The Empowered Physique

Sculpt Your Body with Precision

By Lee Maasen

Copyright © 2023 Lee Maasen

All rights reserved. No part of this publication may be reproduced, distributed, or transmitted in any form or by any means, including photocopying, recording, or other electronic or mechanical methods, without prior written permission of the publisher, except in the case of brief quotations embodied in critical review and certain other noncommercial uses permitted by the copyright law. For permission request, write to the publisher, addressed "Attention: Copyright Permissions" at the email address below.

Email: info@elumethod.com

For more information visit: www.elumethod.com

Disclaimer: This book is for information purposes only. Although the author has made every effort to ensure the information in this book was correct at press time, the author does not assume and hereby disclaims any liability to any party for any loss, damage, or disruption caused by the book. The author and /or distributors are not responsible for any adverse effects resulting from the use of the suggestions outlined in this program.

Table of Contents

Intro: to ELU METHOD

Chapter 1: The Calorie Code

Chapter 2: Powering Up With Protein

Chapter 3: Weights Wins at Metabolic Health

Chapter 4: The Fasting Advantage

Chapter 5: Unveiling the Sweet Deception

Chapter 6: The Regeneration Game

Chapter 7: The Sunshine Vitamin

Chapter 8: Empowered Physique

Dedication

To all the unwavering supporters who have been by my side throughout this incredible journey, this book is dedicated to you.

To my famly, whose love and encouragement have been the foundation of my strength. Thank you for always believing in me and standing beside me, evene when the path seemed daunting.

To you friends, who have been my pillars of support, offering words of motivation and cheering me on every step of the way. Your unwavering friendship has been an invaluable source of inspiration.

To the countless individuals who have shared their stories, struggles, and triumphs with me, thank you for entrusting me with your experiences. Your openness and trust have fuled my determination to make a positive impact in your lives.

To my mentors and coaches, whose guidance and expertise have shaped my understanding and enriched my knowledge. Your wisdom and belief in my potential have been instrumental in my growth.

To the readers of this book, your curiosity and thirst for knowledge have motivated me to share my insights and experiences. Your support and engagement have inspired me to continually strive for excellence.

This book is a testament to the power of collective encouragement and support. May it inspire and empower you to chase your dreams, overcome challenges, and create a life fulfullment.

With gratitude,
Lee

Introduction to ELU METHOD

"4 Essential Elements of Success"

Caloric Balance: Finding The Healthy Deficit
Protein Consumption: Prioritizing Protein Amount
Strength Emphasis: Weightlifting Strength Focus
Morning Fast: Intermittent Fasting for 4-6 Hours

Welcome to the **ELU METHOD**- a comprehensive approach designed to elevate your fitness journey to new heights. Within these pages, you will discover the essential elements of success that will guide you towards achieving your health and wellness goals.

Essential Element #1: Healthy Caloric Deficit forms the foundation of the Enhanced Lifting Fitness System. By understanding the importance of achieving a sustainable caloric deficit, you will learn how to effectively manage your energy intake and expenditure to support sustainable weight loss or maintenance.

Essential Element #2: Proper Protein Consumption takes center stage in our approach. Prioritizing adequate protein consumption will unlock the key to muscle growth, repair, and overall body composition. Learn how to optimize your protein intake and harness its power to support your fitness goals.

Essential Element #3: Strength Emphasis lies at the heart of our exercise philosophy. With weightlifting as the primary focus, you will uncover the transformative benefits of resistance training. From building lean muscle to increasing strength and boosting metabolism, embrace the power of strength training as the cornerstone of your fitness routine.

Essential Element #4: Morning Fast introduces you to the concept of zero-calorie intermittent fasting. Discover the potential benefits of fasting for 4-6 hours in the morning, allowing your body to tap into its fat stores and optimize your metabolism. Learn how to implement this powerful strategy into your daily routine to further enhance your results.

ELU METHOD is your guide to unlocking your true potential, revolutionizing your approach to fitness, and achieving the results you desire. Whether you are a beginner or a seasoned fitness enthusiast, this book will provide you with the knowledge, tools, and guidance to transform your body and elevate your overall well-being.

Get ready to embark on a transformative journey as we delve into the Essential Elements of Success. Together, we will sculpt your physique, enhance your strength, and unlock a new level of fitness prowess. Let the Enhanced Fitness System be your trusted companion on the path to greatness.

Chapter 1: The Calorie Code

Using Total Daily Energy Expenditure(TDEE) and the Mifflin St. Jeor Equation for Weight Loss.

In your journey towards a healthier, fitter self, the first stop is understanding the role of calories in our body and how managing them effectively leads to sustainable weight loss. This chapter demystifies the concept of Total Daily Energy Expenditure (TDEE) and introduces the Mifflin St. Jeor equation, a powerful tool for calculating your precise caloric needs.

Understanding Calories and TDEE

Every activity we perform, from intense workouts to simply breathing, requires energy. This energy comes from the food we consume, which is measured in units called calories.

TDEE is an acronym for Total Daily Energy Expenditure. This is the total number of calories you burn in a day, accounting for your basal metabolic rate, physical activity, and the energy used to digest and absorb food.

Importance of Staying within Calorie Limits

Our body weight is essentially a balance of the calories we consume and the calories we burn. Eating more calories than your TDEE results in weight gain as the excess calories are stored as fat. Conversely, eating fewer calories than your TDEE leads to weight loss as your body burns stored fat to meet its energy requirements.

Maintaining a calorie deficit—eating fewer calories than your TDEE—is the key to weight loss. However, it's important that this deficit is sustainable. An overly aggressive calorie deficit can lead to hormonal imbalances, nutrient deficiencies, and excessive muscle loss. It can also increase feelings of hunger, making the diet difficult or impossible to stick to long term.

Creating a Healthy Caloric Deficit

For people needing to lose 20 pounds of fat or less, a sustainable calorie deficit is between 200-500 calories less than their TDEE. For obese individuals who need to lose 20 pounds of fat or more can have a higher calorie deficit of 1,000. This provides a steady rate of weight loss without drastic changes to your lifestyle or eating habits.

Listening to your body's hunger cues is important. If you find yourself becoming ravenous, it might be a sign that your calorie deficit is too large and you need to increase your calorie intake. Remember, sustainable weight loss is a marathon, not a sprint.

The Power of Consistency

One of the most effective strategies for weight loss is eating the same meals every day for the first 1-2 weeks. This approach helps create a routine and reduces the number of decisions you need to make about food, making it easier to stick to your calorie goals. This is the first "non-negotiable" for weight loss—establish a sustainable, healthy caloric deficit and stick to it for at least three months.

Let's Find Your Total Daily Energy Expenditure (TDEE)

Your TDEE is the total number of calories you burn in a day - accounting for your base metabolism, the food you eat, and your physical activity level. Knowing your TDEE is key for effective weight management.

Mifflin St. Jeor Equation

The Mifflin St. Jeor equation is a popular method to estimate your Basal Metabolic Rate (BMR) - the number of calories your body needs to perform essential functions like breathing, circulating blood, and regulating body temperature. *Let's put it into action:*

For men: BMR = 10 x weight(kg) + 6.25 x height(cm) - 5 x age(y) + 5

For women: BMR = 10 x weight(kg) + 6.25 x height(cm) - 5 x age(y) - 161

Once you have your BMR, you can calculate your TDEE by multiplying your BMR by your physical activity level, which is tySedentary (little to no exercise): BMR x 1.2

Lightly active *(light exercise/sports 1-3 days/week): BMR x 1.375*

Moderately active *(moderate exercise/sports 3-5 days/week): BMR x 1.55*

Very active *(hard exercise/sports 6-7 days a week): BMR x 1.725*

Super active *(very hard exercise/physical job & exercise 2x/day): BMR x 1.9*

My TDEE and Step by Step Instructions

I weigh a 190lb (86.2kg) a male, 6ft (183cm) tall, 30 years old, and I workout four times a week, achieving 8,000 steps a day.. You would classify myself as 'moderately active'.Most people believe they are more active than they actually are. Using the Mifflin St. Jeor equation, we'd calculate my BMR and TDEE as follows:

BMR = 10 x 86.2 + 6.25 x 183 - 5 x 30 + 5 = 1832.5 calories/day

BMR or Basil Metabolic Rate is the amount of calories that is required for your bodily functions to continue working properly to keep your body self operating and alive. For example I could lay in bed all day not moving a muscle and my body will burn 1,832 calories. BMR number is indicating by how metabolic our bodies are by how much muscle mass x fat mass we have. Brown fat is also a metabolic fat that increases our BMR and brown fat is developed by cold adaptation so adding cold showers and cold plunges into your routine will also increase your metabolism.

MY TDEE = 1832.5 x 1.55 = 2839.9 calories/day

To achieve a healthy, sustainable caloric deficit for weight loss, I would aim to consume around 80-90% of my TDEE, which would equate to approximately 2,272 - 2556 calories/day. My healthy caloric intake each day will be between 2,272 - 2,556 which will keep all of my metabolic hormones in check which we will discuss in a later chapter.

Chapter 2: Powering Up With Protein

Your Optimal Protein Intake, The History of Human Food, and Health Benefits of Red Meat

In our last chapter, we discovered the key to weight loss - maintaining a sustainable caloric deficit. However, not all calories are created equal. In this chapter, we'll find your optimal daily protein requirements and delve into the world of protein - a crucial macronutrient, particularly important when we're working towards weight loss and overall health, How human food has changed in the course of history, and the health benefits of eating red meat.

The Power of Protein

The connection between protein and weight loss is something that has been extensively studied, and there's a growing body of evidence supporting the idea that a higher protein diet can indeed aid in weight loss efforts. Here's why:

Appetite Control: Protein is highly satiating, meaning it helps you feel fuller for longer. This is because protein reduces levels of ghrelin, the hormone that stimulates hunger, and increases levels of peptide YY, a hormone that helps you feel satiated. By controlling your appetite, you're less likely to overeat or reach for unhealthy snacks.

Increased Metabolic Rate: Eating protein can boost your metabolism due to the thermic effect of food (TEF), which is the energy required to digest, absorb, and process nutrients. Protein has a higher TEF than carbs or fat, meaning you burn more calories digesting protein than other macronutrients.

Muscle Preservation: When losing weight, it's important to target fat loss while preserving muscle mass. Consuming enough protein can support muscle growth and maintenance, especially when combined with resistance training or weight lifting. Having higher muscle mass will help to increase your resting metabolic rate, allowing you to burn more calories, even while at rest.

Blood Sugar Regulation: Protein helps to slow digestion, which can help regulate your blood sugar levels. This is important as it can help to prevent spikes and crashes in blood sugar, which can lead to feelings of hunger and cravings for unhealthy foods.

Calculating Your Protein Needs

If you're looking to lose weight eating higher protein becomes even more important. The lower the calories go the higher the protein consumption needs to become.. Some experts suggest consuming between 0.65-0.85 x times your body weight in grams of protein per day. For example, I weigh 190 pounds, that would equate to approximately 123.5 - 161.5 grams of protein per day.

190 x .65 = 123.5

190 x .85 + 161.5

I always recommend people to eat .85 x body weight because the older we get the more protein we need to consume.

The Role of Red Meat

Red meat is often misunderstood in nutritional circles. Red meat is a rich source of high-quality protein and other key nutrients. Here are some benefits of eating red meat:

High-Quality Protein: Red meat is a source of high-quality protein, which contains all the essential amino acids required by the body. Protein is crucial for maintaining and building muscle mass, which is important for overall health, particularly as we age.

Rich in Nutrients: Red meat is nutrient-dense, providing a wealth of vitamins and minerals. These include B vitamins, particularly B12 which is not found in plant foods, as well as iron, zinc, and selenium.

Supports Muscle Health: Red meat has direct importance of skeletal muscle for health and longevity. Red meat, with its high protein content and rich array of nutrients, supports the health and maintenance of muscle.

There is a long list of real doctors advocating for red meat but here are a few:

Dr. Gabrielle Lyon: As a functional medicine physician, Dr. Lyon supports the consumption of high-quality, nutrient-dense proteins, including red meat. She often emphasizes the role of muscle-centric medicine, highlighting the importance of protein for maintaining muscle health and overall wellbeing.

Dr. Paul Saladino: Known for his advocacy of the "Carnivore Diet," Dr. Saladino supports the consumption of red meat as a primary source of nutrition. He argues that animal foods, especially organ meats, can provide all the necessary nutrients the human body needs.

Dr. Ken Berry: A family physician, Dr. Berry promotes a low-carb, high-fat diet that includes red meat. He often emphasizes the potential benefits of a ketogenic diet for weight loss and the management of various health conditions.

Dr. Shawn Baker: An orthopedic surgeon, Dr. Baker is another advocate for the "Carnivore Diet." He believes that a diet centered around animal products, including red meat, can promote health and fitness.

The history of humans eating red meat dates back to the dawn of our species. It has played a pivotal role in our evolution and development. Let's dive a bit deeper:

Control of Fire: The discovery of fire, which happened around 1-1.5 million years ago(as far as we know), revolutionized human diets. Cooking not only made meat more bioavailable for out health.This extra energy likely contributed to the continued growth of our brains.

Easier Digestion: Cooking partially breaks down proteins and collagen in meat, making it softer and easier to chew and digest. This allows the digestive enzymes in our body to access and break down the proteins more efficiently, thereby increasing the proportion of protein that the body can absorb and use.

Increased Nutrient Availability: Cooking also helps to make certain nutrients in meat more available. For instance, the iron in cooked meat is more readily absorbed than the iron in raw meat. Similarly, cooking also aids in the absorption of other important nutrients, such as vitamins B6 and B12.

Kills Harmful Bacteria: Cooking meat at the right temperature kills harmful bacteria and parasites that can cause foodborne illnesses. Some of these pathogens can interfere with the body's ability to absorb nutrients from food, so eliminating them through cooking also contributes to increased nutrient availability.

Agricultural Revolution: With the advent of agriculture around 10,000 years ago, human diets began to shift towards more plant-based foods. However, domestication of animals also meant that meat remained a crucial part of the diet for many societies. Some people argue that this shift has had negative implications for human health, as our bodies didn't have sufficient time, evolutionarily speaking, to adapt to efficiently processing these new food sources. Here are some reasons why:

Gluten and other Antinutrients: Many grains contain substances like gluten and lectins that can be difficult for some people to digest. These substances can cause inflammation and damage to the lining of the gut, especially in individuals with celiac disease or gluten intolerance.

High in Carbohydrates: Grains are high in carbohydrates, and overconsumption can lead to issues like insulin resistance, obesity, and diabetes, especially when the grains are highly processed and stripped of their fiber and nutrients.

Gut Health: Modern grains, especially refined ones, lack beneficial fibers and nutrients that support a healthy gut microbiome. Poor gut health has been linked to a variety of health issues, from mental health problems to autoimmune diseases.

Industrial Era: The industrialization of the 19th and 20th centuries transformed mass eating recommendations. The industrial era marked significant changes in the way food was produced and consumed. As technologies advanced, food processing became more widespread, and many foods underwent significant changes in their composition, often for the worse. *Here's how the rise of processed foods has had implications for our health:*

High in Added Sugars and Unhealthy Fats: Many processed foods are high in added sugars and unhealthy fats, including trans fats and saturated fats. Consuming too much of these can increase the risk of obesity, heart disease, type 2 diabetes, and certain types of cancer.

High in Sodium: Processed foods often contain high levels of sodium, which can contribute to high blood pressure and increase the risk of heart disease and stroke.

Low in Nutrients: Processed foods are often lower in essential nutrients than whole foods. They can be stripped of valuable fiber, vitamins, and minerals during processing. The result is what's often referred to as "empty calories" - foods with high caloric content but low nutritional value.

Artificial Ingredients: Many processed foods contain a plethora of artificial ingredients, such as preservatives, colorants, flavorings, and texturants. Some of these substances have been linked to health problems.

Overconsumption: Processed foods are often designed to be hyper-palatable, leading to overeating and associated health problems like obesity and metabolic health. The high levels of sugar and fat in these foods can also lead to changes in the brain that promote addiction-like eating behaviors.

Impacts on Gut Health: The lack of fiber and nutrients in processed foods can have negative impacts on the gut microbiota, potentially contributing to a range of health problems from inflammatory bowel disease to mental health issues.

In summary, we as a whole have completely switched which types of food we are eating from whole healthy fat based meals to highly processed sugar meals and our metabolic syndrome or metabolic switch no longer works. The *"Metabolic Switch"* is our bodies ability to switch over from burning sugar as fuel and to burning fat as fuel. Unfortunately roughly 80% and soon to be 90% of the United States population is suffering with this problem that can easily be reversed with this program.

Chapter 3: Weights Wins at Metabolic Health

Resistance Training versus Cardio for Improved Metabolic Health and Body Composition

In our journey towards a healthier body, it's critical to understand the role of resistance training versus cardio. While both forms of exercise have their place in a balanced fitness routine, understanding their impact on our bodies can help us make more informed decisions about our fitness strategy.

Resistance training is key when it comes to improving body composition. When we perform resistance exercises, we essentially break down our muscle fibers. Our bodies then work to repair these fibers, and in doing so, they build larger and stronger muscles. This process not only aids in muscle growth but also in elevating our resting metabolic rate - the rate at which our bodies burn calories at rest. This is because muscle tissue is a metabolically active tissue and fat tissue is not. This means the more muscle mass we have, the more calories we burn throughout the day, even when we're not exercising.

Progressive overload is a fundamental principle of strength training and fitness, referring to the gradual increase in stress placed upon the body during exercise. It's how you get stronger and build muscle over time. In the context of a caloric deficit and weight loss, it becomes even more crucial. In a caloric deficit, your body is using more energy than it's receiving from food. When combined with resistance training, it will encourage your body to use stored energy or fat as fuel while preserving or even building muscle in the process.

Here's how Progressive Overload works:

Start with a manageable load: Begin with a weight that you can lift with proper form for your desired number of repetitions.

Incrementally increase the load: As your strength improves, gradually add more weight. This could be as little as a 2.5lb increase from one session to the next.

Consistency is key: The idea is to make small, consistent increases over time. This could be increasing the weight you lift, the number of repetitions you complete, or the number of sets you perform.

Track your progress: Keep a log of your workouts, noting the exercises, weights, sets, and reps you've done. This way, you can see your progress and know when it's time to increase the challenge.

Remember, the goal isn't to lift as heavy as possible right off the bat, but to increase your strength gradually and consistently while maintaining good form. This approach can help you retain muscle mass while losing weight, leading to a leaner, stronger physique over time.

Finally, it's important to understand that in a caloric deficit, progress may be slower compared to being in a caloric surplus, and that's okay because we are focusing on targeting fat loss. However if you do train hard enough while eating a proper protein amount you can build muscle even while eating in a caloric deficit.

Cardio, on the other hand, while excellent for cardiovascular health and endurance, can present some challenges when it comes to weight loss. The human body is an adaptive machine, always striving for balance. So, when we burn calories through cardio, our bodies often respond by increasing our appetite to replace those burned calories - a phenomenon known as the energy balance theory. This can make weight management tricky if not properly balanced with a healthy diet and resistance training.

For example high-intensity cardio such as Orange Theory, F45 Training, Barry's Bootcamp, Crossfit, and Soul Cycle workouts do not focus on building strength or muscle. These companies focus on burning as many calories as possible which causes massive increase in appetite and massive stress on the body.

The stress hormone is called "Cortisol". And elevated cortisol levels in the body will force the body to hold on to fat and causes many people to have that "skinny fat" look they are trying to avoid. Unfortunately when our bodies train in heart rate zones 3, 4, and 5 our bodies will begin to lose muscle. This is because our body will pull energy(calories) out of muscle tissue and not fat tissue.

For example if an individual works out at Orange theory and loses 10 lbs and looks "skinny fat". This is because they have lost 5lbs of fat and 5lbs of muscle. This is what happens in the higher heart rate zones and why the Empowered Physique Protocol does not prescribe hard cardio workouts. We recommend people to stay in Zone 2 cardio and walk 8,000 steps a day. We will discuss these details later in the book.

Training in the higher heart rate zones cause a lot stress(Cortisol) on the body and prolonged elevation of cortisol can lead to undesirable effects, including weight gain and weight loss resistance. High cortisol wil promote fat storage particularly in the abdominal area. It will also suppress other hormones, such as testosterone, which plays a crucial role in muscle growth and strength, fat distribution, and overall wellbeing for both men and women. A quick side note, testosterone and dopamine act as cousins. If testosterone is down that inevitably means dopamine is down as well.

For the purposes of the ELU METHOD, we are aiming to stay within **Zone 2**, 60-70% of Max Heart Rate(MHR), during cardio activities, as this zone promotes fat burning without raising cortisol levels. This heart rate zone even increases mitochondrial health, recovery, and increases serotonin.

To find your max target heart rate subtract your age from 220. Aim to exercise within 60-70% of that number. For the majority of people, this zone corresponds to a heart rate range of approximately 120-145 beats per minute. Training in this zone encourages the body to effectively burn fat for fuel, aiding in weight loss and overall health improvement. While the intensity in Zone 2 may be considered relatively light to moderate - typically allowing for comfortable conversation during exercise - its impact should not be underestimated.

By regularly incorporating Zone 2 cardio exercises, such as brisk walking(8,000 steps per day), light jogging, or cycling, into their fitness regimen, individuals can optimally balance calorie burning, cardiovascular health, and the control of stress hormones like cortisol that we are focusing on keeping low.. It's the perfect sweet spot for sustainable, long-term fitness progress.

Here are your 5 Essential Heart Rate Zones:

Zone 1 - Very Light (50-60% of Maximum Heart Rate [MHR]):

This is essentially the warm-up and cool-down stage, involving light activities such as stretching and slow walking. It's great for recovery and getting your body ready for more intense exercise.

Zone 2 - Light (60-70% of MHR):

This is where light cardio comes in, such as brisk walking or light cycling. This zone is perfect for improving basic endurance and fat burning. It's also the optimal zone for those who are beginning their fitness journey or want to focus solely on training their heart and lungs.

Zone 3 - Moderate (70-80% of MHR):

This is a more intense cardio zone, typically reached during steady-state exercises like jogging or swimming. There are no benefits to zone 3 cardio that zone 2 cardio doesn't already provide. Zone 3 increases injury risk, increases cortisol, and the body starts pulling calories out of the muscle because this zone starts to "lactate" or have the burning sensation.

Zone 4 - Hard (80-90% of MHR):

In this zone, you're running hard or doing high-intensity interval training (HIIT). It's great for improving your anaerobic capacity and threshold. This heart rate zone should always be done properly and it is not advised to complete multiple times a week. This zone also has a high risk of injury, increases appetite, and spikes cortisol.

Zone 5 - Maximum (90-100% of MHR):

This zone is the most intense, achieved during sprinting or other all-out efforts. It's excellent for improving speed and power. However, this zone should only be visited briefly and infrequently, as it stresses your body the most. This zone has a very high risk of injury but also does provide high reward for those who execute this zone training properly. This zone does build muscle but is absolutely lung busting and not sustainable without a properly plan for recovery.

For the purposes of the Enhanced Physique Protocol, we are aiming to stay at Zone 2 (60-70% of MHR) during cardio activities, as this zone promotes fat burning without excessively raising cortisol levels.

You can do your easy cardio days alternating with your weight lifting or resistance training days.

Here's a simple yet effective Empowered Physique full-body workout plan for a beginner that you can do 3 times a week. As a beginner, it's important to focus on learning the correct form and technique for each exercise to prevent injuries. Also, remember to begin each session with a warm-up and finish with a cool-down.

Warm-Up

Aim for around 5-10 minutes of light cardio such as brisk walking or jogging on a treadmill.

Day 1
1. Low Incline DB Press: 3 sets of 10-12 reps
2. Reverse Grip Lat Pulldown: 3 sets of 10-12 reps
3. Squats: 3 sets of 10-12 reps
4. Dumbbell Lateral Raises: 3 sets of 10-12 reps
5. Cable Face Pulls: 3 sets of 10-12 reps
6. Cable Preacher Curl: 3 sets of 10-12 reps

Day 2
1. Seated Dumbbell Shoulder Press: 3 sets of 10-12 reps
2. Leg Press: 3 sets of 10-12 reps
3. Weighted Hyperextension:: 3 sets of 10-12 reps

4. Seated Cable Row: 3 sets of 10-12 reps
5. Dumbbell Lunges: 3 sets of 10-12 reps per leg
6. Cable Tricep Pressdown: 3 sets of 10-12 reps

Day 3
1. Chest to Wall Hold: 3 sets of 20-30 second hold
2. Reverse Lunge: 3 sets of 10-12 rep/each
3. Lying Leg Curls: 3 sets of 10-12 reps
4. Wide-Grip Lat Pulldown: 3 sets of 10-12 reps
5. Chest Supported Dumbbell Front Raise: 3 sets of 10-12 reps
6. Cable Hammer Curls: 3 sets of 10-12 reps

Cool-Down

Finish your workout with a 5-10 minute cool-down period. This could include stretches or light cardio.

Please note: Listen to your body and adjust the weights, repetitions, or sets as necessary. It's better to lift lighter weights with proper form than heavier weights with poor form. You can increase the weight as you get stronger. And, always consult with a healthcare provider before starting any new exercise program.

Remember to always prioritize the weight lighting or resistance training workouts over cardio workouts. We want to build muscle and strength to shape out bodies for long-term health and body composition results. Building muscle and strength increases our metabolism and maintains muscle mass even while in a caloric deficit. Extreme cardio will increase our appetite making it much harder to stick to the diet plan and will also spike stress in the body which will lower testosterone and promote our body to hold on to fat.

Chapter 4: The Fasting Advantage

Harnessing the Fat-Burning and Health Benefits of Intermittent Fasting

Most of us were brought up with the age-old mantra, "Breakfast is the most important meal of the day." However, a growing body of research suggests that delaying the first meal of the day, a practice known as intermittent fasting, will have a powerful impact on our body composition and overall health.

Intermittent fasting isn't a diet; it's a pattern of eating. It doesn't change what you eat, but when you eat. By simply shifting our eating window, we can tap into our body's innate ability to burn fat and improve our health markers.

The practice of fasting and consuming zero calories for the first 4-6 hours upon waking puts our body into a state of 'fat-burning' mode. But how does this work? Well, when we consume food, our body spends a few hours processing the nutrients and generating energy. During this period, our body is in a "fed" state and it's impossible for our body to burn fat because insulin levels are high.

However, after this post-meal period, our body enters a state of fasting. Insulin levels drop and the body begins to use stored fat for energy. Therefore, by extending the overnight fasting period and pushing the first meal of the day out a few hours, we capitalize on the body's natural fat-burning mechanism.

Intermittent fasting also has several health benefits. Research has shown it can help reduce inflammation, improve heart health, and even enhance brain function. Moreover, it simplifies your day and can free up time.

There's also an important psychological benefit. Many people find that intermittent fasting helps them break free from the shackles of constant eating, food cravings, and sugar highs and lows. It puts you back in control of your appetite.

But as with everything related to our health, it's important to listen to our bodies. If you try intermittent fasting and find it's not for you, that's okay. There are many paths to health and wellness, and the best approach is always the one that fits with your lifestyle and makes you feel your best.

If you are new to intermittent fasting there are several strategies you can use to make the transition easier:

Increase Salt Intake: Salt is a key electrolyte that is often flushed out of our bodies when we begin fasting. Consuming a bit more salt can help reduce the symptoms of the 'keto flu', a common side effect of transitioning to a fasting lifestyle, which includes headaches, fatigue, and nausea. You can add a pinch of high-quality sea salt to your water or even just place it directly on your tongue.

Use BCAA and EAA Supplements: Branched-chain amino acids (BCAAs) and essential amino acids (EAAs) are helpful during fasting periods, especially for those who exercise. They can help preserve muscle tissue and provide a source of energy during your workout, all without breaking your fast. Just make sure to look for a supplement without added sugars or calories.

Stay Hydrated: This might seem like a no-brainer, but it's surprising how often the sensation of hunger is actually your body telling you it's thirsty. Make sure you're drinking plenty of water throughout your fast.

Keep Busy: One of the best ways to combat hunger during a fast is to distract yourself. If you're busy, you'll have less time to think about food. This could be a great time to delve into a project you've been meaning to tackle, or to engage in an activity that keeps your mind engaged.

Gradual Progression: If you're new to intermittent fasting, it may be easier to gradually increase your fasting window rather than jumping straight into a full 16-hour fast. You could start with a 12-hour fast, then slowly increase your fasting window by 30 minutes to an hour every few days until you reach your goal.

Listen to Your Body: It's normal to feel a little hungry during a fast, but if you're feeling dizzy, faint, or excessively hungry, it might be a sign that you need to break your fast. Listen to your body and adjust your fasting schedule as needed.

Historical Perspective

Our ancestors often fasted out of necessity, when food was scarce. They had to hunt and gather food, and there would be times when they couldn't find anything to eat, resulting in involuntary periods of fasting. Their bodies adapted to this cycle of feast and famine. Research suggests that our bodies are still biologically adapted for this type of eating pattern, which is part of the reason intermittent fasting can have such profound health benefits.

Fasting is a powerful tool that can stimulate a variety of beneficial physiological changes in your body. Two of the key benefits of fasting include the promotion of ketosis and the preservation of muscle mass:

Ketosis is a metabolic state that occurs when your body starts using fat as its primary source of fuel, rather than carbohydrates. Normally, the body relies on glucose for energy, which is derived from the carbohydrates we eat. When you fast, your body exhausts its glucose stores and starts breaking down fat to produce molecules known as ketones. *Using ketones as a source of energy has a number of potential health benefits:*

Weight Loss: By using fat stores for energy, your body actively burns fat, which will promote weight loss.

Improved Brain Function: Research suggests that ketones are a more efficient energy source for the brain than glucose, and will improve cognitive function.

Reduced Inflammation: Ketosis will also reduce inflammation, a key driver of many chronic diseases.

Improved Insulin Sensitivity: Fasting and the resultant ketosis will improve insulin sensitivity, which can be particularly beneficial for people with insulin resistance or type 2 diabetes.

Preservation of Muscle Mass also occurs when ketones are present. When you're trying to lose weight, it's important to ensure that you're only losing fat, not muscle. *Contrary to popular belief, fasting doesn't lead to muscle loss, but rather it can actually help preserve muscle mass:*

Human Growth Hormone (HGH): Fasting stimulates the production of HGH, a hormone that plays a crucial role in muscle growth and recovery.

Protein Conservation: After the initial stages of fasting, your body enters a state of protein conservation, breaking down mostly fat for energy and sparing your muscles.

Resistance Training: Combining fasting with resistance training can be particularly effective. The increased HGH from fasting can enhance the muscle-building effects of resistance exercise.

In conclusion, the practice of fasting is a potent catalyst for reaching ketosis, burning fat, and preserving muscle. This all leads to an improved overall health and well-being.

Chapter 5: Unveiling the Sweet Deception

Mastering Insulin Regulation and Unmasking Hidden Sugars

In this crucial chapter, we delve into the details of insulin regulation and shine a light on the hidden sugars that lurk in the depths of ingredient lists. By understanding the impact of insulin on our bodies and learning to identify and avoid hidden sugars, we unlock the key to maintaining stable energy levels, optimizing weight management, and promoting overall health.

When insulin is present, it will turn off the production and release of certain hormones in the body. These hormones that insulin turns are are:

Glucagon: Insulin and glucagon work in opposition to regulate blood sugar levels. When insulin levels rise, glucagon secretion decreases. Glucagon is responsible for stimulating the liver to release stored glucose into the bloodstream, thereby increasing blood sugar levels. Insulin stops the release of glucagon, preventing the liver from releasing additional glucose. Glucagon plays a critical role in signaling the liver to start the production of ketones and promote fat burning. Ketones are molecules produced by the liver when glucose availability is limited, such as during periods of fasting or low carbohydrate intake. They serve as an alternative fuel source for the body, particularly the brain and muscles.

Growth Hormone: Insulin will suppress the release of growth hormone (GH) from the pituitary gland. Growth hormone is essential for tissue repair, muscle growth, and overall body development. Elevated insulin levels, particularly in response to high carbohydrate meals, will inhibit the release of growth hormone, impacting muscle-building and repair processes.

Lipolysis Hormones: Insulin inhibits the release of lipolysis hormones, such as glucagon, adrenaline (epinephrine), and norepinephrine. These hormones play a crucial role in the breakdown of stored fat (lipolysis) to release fatty acids into the bloodstream for energy utilization. When insulin is present, lipolysis is suppressed, and the body's ability to access and burn stored fat as a fuel source is diminished.

Leptin: Insulin will influence the production and signaling of leptin, a hormone produced by fat cells. Leptin plays a role in regulating appetite, metabolism, and energy balance. When insulin levels are consistently elevated, it can interfere with leptin signaling, potentially contributing to leptin resistance and disrupted appetite control.

So with all these hormone changes it is extremely important to keep insulin down as much as possible through out the day. It is also important to learn what the hidden sugars are that companies will hide on the back in the ingredients list that still spike our insulin.

When we consume products containing artificial sugars, such as zero-calorie sweeteners, the sweet taste on our taste buds signals the brain to expect an influx of glucose.

In response, the pancreas releases insulin to help process and metabolize the anticipated rise in blood sugar. This insulin release can occur even when there are no actual calories present in the artificial sweeteners.

Insulin response to artificial sugars will interrupt the fat-burning process and definitely impact ketosis. Insulin promotes the uptake and storage of glucose, inhibiting the breakdown of stored fats and the production of ketone bodies. Even without consuming actual calories, the release of insulin will temporarily shift the body's metabolism away from fat burning and hinder the maintenance of a state of ketosis.

Therefore, it is essential to be mindful of consuming products with artificial sugars, especially if the goal is to maintain fat burning or stay in a state of ketosis. While these sweeteners may not contribute to calorie intake, they will still impact insulin levels and interfere with metabolic processes associated with fat burning.

To support fat burning and ketosis, it is recommended to minimize the consumption of artificial sweeteners and focus on whole, unprocessed foods. This allows for a more balanced and natural approach to nutrition, while reducing the potential for unintended insulin responses that wil hinder fat burning and ketosis.

Here is a list of the "Hidden Sugars" on the back on your grocery ingredient list that is keeping you from fat burning:

1. Brown Sugar
2. Dextrose
3. Glucose
4. Honey
5. Maltose
6. Raw Sugar
7. Sucanat(pure dried sugar can juice)
8. Barley Malt
9. Corn Sweetener
10. Fructose
11. High-Fructose Corn Syrup
12. Invert Sugar

13. Malt Syrup
14. Sucrose
15. Brown Rice Syrup
16. Corn Syrup
17. Fruit Juice Concentrates
18. Processed White Sugar Lactose
19. Molasses
20. Syrup
21. Turbinado
22. Agave Nectar

Now, armed with the knowledge of hidden sugars cleverly concealed on ingredient lists, you possess the power to maintain ketosis and accelerate fat burning. By staying vigilant and mindful of the deceptive tactics employed by companies, you can make informed choices that keep you on track towards your goals. Avoiding hidden sugars allows you to optimize your body's ability to burn fat and experience the full benefits of a ketogenic lifestyle. With this newfound awareness, you can confidently navigate the world of food labels, ensuring that you stay in ketosis and unlock the accelerated fat-burning potential within you.

They key to losing weight is being able to control insulin. *Here is a quick reminder on the topics of this chapter because knowledge is extremely significant.*

The Insulin Connection

When insulin is present in our bodies, the process of burning fat becomes significantly hindered. Insulin, a hormone secreted by the pancreas, is responsible for regulating our blood sugar levels. Its primary role is to facilitate the uptake of glucose into our cells for energy or storage. However, when insulin levels are elevated, our body's ability to tap into fat stores and burn stored fat is compromised. Also when insulin is present it also turns off all the other metabolic hormones because it is such a powerful hormone.

The Impact of Hidden Sugars

Hidden sugars can wreak havoc on our bodies, leading to weight gain, energy crashes, and increased risk of chronic diseases. There are absolute detrimental effects of excessive sugar intake and by understanding the relationship between hidden sugars and insulin spikes, we gain insight into how these sneaky ingredients will disrupt our energy levels, hinder weight loss efforts, and contribute to long-term health complications.

Strategies for Sugar Awareness

Equipped with the knowledge of insulin regulation and hidden sugars, it is important to explore practical strategies to keep our insulin levels in check and minimize our consumption of hidden sugars. From mindful grocery shopping to meal planning, recipe modifications, and conscious choices that support our goals for improved health and body composition.

Chapter 6: The Regeneration Game

Importance of Sleep, Hormones, and Dopamine

Welcome to the fifth chapter of our journey, where we get into the intricate world of sleep and hormones and their impact on your health and fitness. You might be surprised to learn just how important our nightly rest, our hormone balance, and our dopamine levels intertwine, contributing to our overall well-being and fitness results.

First, let's consider sleep. It isn't merely a time for our minds to check out from the hustle and bustle of the day. While we sleep, our bodies are hard at work, restoring, repairing, and rebuilding. During the deep stages of sleep, our bodies release growth hormone, a powerful substance that repairs tissue, builds muscle, and burns fat. Growth hormone is also the "Anti-Aging" hormone that we lose as we get older. This overnight renovation process is crucial for maintaining our physical health, particularly if we're putting our bodies under the stress of regular exercise.

Now, let's move on to cortisol, often referred to as the 'stress hormone.' Under normal circumstances, cortisol plays a vital role in our bodies. It helps us respond to danger, regulates our metabolism, reduces inflammation, and even has a hand in memory formulation. However, when our bodies are subjected to chronic stress or lack of sleep, cortisol levels can skyrocket. This increase in cortisol can have a series negative effects, including suppressing other hormones, notably testosterone.

Testosterone is a crucial hormone for both men and women. It's linked to muscle mass, bone density, energy levels, and sexual health. However, its role doesn't stop there. There's a direct link between testosterone and dopamine, the neurotransmitter associated with pleasure, motivation, and reward systems in our brain. When testosterone levels drop, dopamine levels can drop as well, leading to feelings of lethargy, low mood, and a lack of motivation.

Now we understand how sleep effects our hormones. We need to optimize our sleep and sleep schedule. This can vary from person to person, as we all have individual needs and lifestyles. However, research shows that certain guidelines promote better sleep quality and overall health.

Consistency: Try to go to bed and wake up at the same time every day, even on weekends. This helps regulate your body's internal clock, known as your circadian rhythm.

Duration: Aim for 7-9 hours of sleep per night. This is the recommended range for adults by sleep experts and is associated with the best health outcomes.

Nightly Routine: Establish a pre-sleep routine to help signal to your body that it's time to wind down and go to sleep. This could involve reading a book, having a hot shower, or doing some light stretching.

Environment: Keep your sleep environment dark, quiet, cool, and comfortable. Consider using earplugs or an eye mask if necessary, and make sure your mattress and pillows are comfortable.

Limit Exposure to Blue Light: The blue light from screens (phones, computers, TV) will interfere with your body's production of melatonin, the hormone that regulates sleep. Try to turn off these devices at least an hour before bed or wear blue light blocking glasses.

Limit Napping: While short power naps can be beneficial, long or irregular napping during the day can negatively affect your sleep.

Be Mindful of Food and Drink: Avoid large meals, caffeine, and alcohol close to bedtime. This will disrupt your sleep cycle and drinking alcohol will block the release of growth hormone altogether.

Sleep is truly the unsung hero of a healthy lifestyle, and it plays an incredibly important role in body composition and overall health. Here's why:

Weight Management: Lack of sleep can disrupt the balance of key hormones that control appetite. When you're sleep deprived, you may feel hungrier and find it harder to feel full, leading to overeating and weight gain.

Muscle Recovery and Growth: Sleep is the time your body repairs and grows muscle tissue. Growth hormone is primarily released during deep sleep. Not getting enough sleep will limit this process and can slow down your fitness gains.

Insulin Sensitivity and Metabolism: Sleep helps maintain a healthy balance of the hormones that make you feel hungry (ghrelin) or full (leptin). When you don't get enough sleep, your level of ghrelin goes up and your level of leptin goes down. This makes you feel hungrier than when you're well-rested. Sleep deprivation also impairs glucose metabolism and increases the risk of type 2 diabetes.

Mental Health and Mood: Regular good quality sleep keeps your mind sharp and your mood happy. On the flip side, sleep deprivation is linked with mood disorders like depression and anxiety.

Immune Function: During sleep, your body produces proteins called cytokines, some of which help promote sleep. Certain cytokines need to increase when you have an infection or inflammation, or when you're under stress. Sleep deprivation may decrease production of these protective cytokines, making you more susceptible to illnesses.

Heart Health: Sleep affects processes that keep your heart and blood vessels healthy, including your blood sugar, blood pressure, and inflammation levels. It also plays a vital role in your body's ability to heal and repair your heart and blood vessels, making sleep critical for cardiovascular health.

All in all, you cannot underestimate the power of a good night's sleep. It's not just about feeling rested - sleep is a critical component of maintaining a healthy body, a sharp mind, and an optimal body composition. For anyone looking to improve their health or body composition, assessing and improving sleep quality should be a top priority.

Chapter 7: The Sunshine Vitamin

Importance of Vitamin D for Weight Loss and Overall Health

Vitamin D, often referred to as the 'sunshine vitamin' and plays a crucial role in numerous bodily functions, notably in hormone health and immunity. Its impact on these areas is profound, emphasizing the importance of maintaining adequate Vitamin D levels for overall health.

Hormone Health: Vitamin D is, in fact, not just a vitamin, but a pro-hormone. This means it assists in the creation and function of hormones in the body. It is particularly linked to the production and regulation of insulin, a hormone that helps manage blood glucose levels. Vitamin D enhances the body's sensitivity to insulin, supporting a healthy metabolism and potentially reducing the risk of insulin resistance and type 2 diabetes.

Vitamin D has a significant impact on mood-regulating hormones, including serotonin and dopamine. Research has shown that vitamin D deficiency is linked with mood disorders such as depression, and this highlights the importance of this nutrient for mental health.

Immune System Health: Vitamin D is a powerful immune modulator. It has both anti-inflammatory and immunoregulatory properties, making it crucial for the activation of immune system defenses. Vitamin D is known to enhance the function of immune cells, including T-cells and macrophages, that protect your body from pathogens.

The association between vitamin D and immune function is evident in the prevention of autoimmune diseases and infections. Low levels of vitamin D have been linked to an increased susceptibility to infection, diseases such as multiple sclerosis, and respiratory illnesses.

In addition to these roles, vitamin D is essential for healthy bone formation and calcium absorption in the gut, adding to its list of important functions in the body.

Maintaining adequate levels of vitamin D is not just beneficial, but essential for hormone balance, robust immune health, and overall well-being. While sunlight, certain foods, and supplements can help achieve this, it's important to consult with a healthcare professional for personalized advice, particularly if considering supplements.

Scientific evidence has shown that vitamin D deficiency is prevalent among those with obesity and that higher body fat is associated with lower vitamin D levels. The relationship between vitamin D and body weight may lie in the role of vitamin D in the regulation of fat cells. In lab studies, vitamin D has been found to influence the cells' ability to store or burn fat, impacting weight gain and loss.

Vitamin D also plays a role in our overall health and well-being. Our solar plexus, located in the upper abdomen, acts as the gateway for optimal absorption of this vital nutrient. When sunlight hits our skin, it triggers the production of vitamin D within our bodies. By spending time outdoors and exposing our skin to sunlight, we can ensure that our solar plexus absorbs this essential vitamin efficiently. So step outside, bask in the sun, and let your solar plexus become the portal to optimal vitamin D absorption and radiant well-being.

Chapter 8: Empowered Physique

Unleashing Your Full Potential

In this final chapter, we bring together all the key elements discussed throughout this book to create the ultimate fitness regimen—the Empowered Physique program. Combining the knowledge gained from previous chapters, we will guide you in crafting a personalized plan that optimizes your weight loss, muscle gain, and overall health.

Calculating Your TDEE and Protein Requirements: Begin by revisiting Chapter 1 and Chapter 2. Using the Mifflin St. Jeor equation, calculate your Total Daily Energy Expenditure (TDEE) to determine your optimal caloric intake for weight loss, subtract 200-500 calories or stay within 80-90% of your TDEE.. Consider your protein requirements, ensuring you meet the optimal intake range (.65-.85 x body weight in grams of protein) outlined in Chapter 2, but best results will be at .85 x bodyweight.

Resistance Training for Body Composition: Incorporate resistance training into your routine as discussed in Chapter 3. Design a workout program that targets all major muscle groups, focusing on compound exercises such as squats, deadlifts, bench presses, and rows. Aim to train at least three days a week, progressively increasing the intensity and volume over time. Be sure to avoid intense cardio sessions and keep heart rate in zone 2 which for most people will be between 120-145 bpm. Also it is important to walk 8,000 steps per day for overall health and addional calories burned.

Strategic Fasting and Rest: Leverage the benefits of intermittent fasting outlined in Chapter 4. Implement the practice of fasting for the first 4-6 hours after waking up, allowing your body to tap into fat stores for energy. Balance fasting periods with appropriate rest and recovery to ensure optimal muscle repair and growth.

Prioritize Quality Sleep: Understand the importance of sleep highlighted in Chapter 5. Establish a consistent sleep routine, aiming for 7-9 hours of uninterrupted sleep each night. Create a sleep-friendly environment, minimizing exposure to blue light from electronic devices before bed, and practicing relaxation techniques to promote deep and restorative sleep.

Harness the Power of Vitamin D: Maintain sufficient vitamin D levels as discussed in Chapter 6. Incorporate sunlight exposure when possible and consume vitamin D-rich foods or supplements to support hormone health, immune function, and overall wellbeing.

Personalization and Progression: Tailor your fitness program to suit your individual needs and goals. Track your progress, both in terms of weight loss and strength gains, to ensure you are consistently challenging your body and progressing towards your desired results.

As we reach the final pages of this book, it is important to reflect on the Essential Elements of Success that have been shared with you. Caloric Balance, Proper Protein Consumption, Strength Emphasis, and Morning Fast have formed the pillars of your journey towards an empowered physique and long-term weight loss solution.

"Essential Elements of Success"

Caloric Balance: Finding The Healthy Deficit
Protein Consumption: Prioritizing Protein Amount
Strength Emphasis: Weightlifting Strength Focus
Morning Fast: Intermittent Fasting for 4-6 Hours

By achieving a healthy caloric deficit, you have discovered the power of balancing your energy intake and expenditure. This fundamental principle has allowed you to take control of your body composition and create sustainable changes that will lead to lasting results. You have learned to nourish your body with the right amount of nutrients while being mindful of your energy needs.

Prioritizing adequate protein consumption has been a game-changer in your fitness journey. By understanding the role of protein in muscle growth, repair, and overall body composition, you have unlocked the key to transforming your physique. Through conscious choices and incorporating protein-rich foods into your meals, you have provided your body with the necessary building blocks for success.

Strength Emphasis has revolutionized your approach to exercise. By embracing weightlifting as the main focus of your workouts, you have witnessed the transformative power of resistance training. Building lean muscle, increasing strength, and boosting your metabolism have become your new normal. With each rep and set, you have sculpted a physique that radiates strength and confidence.

The practice of Morning Fast has added another dimension to your fitness journey. By implementing zero-calorie intermittent fasting for 4-6 hours each morning, you have tapped into your body's innate ability to utilize stored fat for energy. This strategic fasting period has not only supported your weight loss goals but has also optimized your metabolism and provided mental clarity to conquer the day ahead.

Now armed with the knowledge and understanding of these Essential Elements of Success, you possess the tools to sustain your empowered physique and long-term weight loss solution. This is not a quick fix or a temporary solution, but a lifestyle that you have embraced wholeheartedly. You have forged a path towards optimal health, vitality, and self-confidence.

As you close this book, remember that you are the author of your own journey. Embrace the power within you, continue to prioritize your health, and let the Essential Elements of Success guide you towards continued growth and fulfillment. May your empowered physique be a testament to your unwavering dedication and commitment to living your best life.

Congratulations on embarking on this transformative path. The world awaits the radiance and strength you will bring. Now, go forth and embrace the empowered physique and the lifelong joy of a healthy, balanced, and fulfilling existence.

With the Essential Elements of Success as your compass, the possibilities are endless. Seize them and create the life you deserve.

Here's to your continued success and a future filled with vitality and confidence!

This is to your Empowered Physique fitness journey

ELU NATION

Thank you

To the incredible individuals who have taken the leap and embarked on a profound journey of self-discovery and transformation, this page is dedicated to you, ELU NATION.

Your commitment to your health and well-being inspires me beyond words. By diving deep into the intricacies of your own physical and mental health, you have shown immense courage and dedication. Your pursuit of excellence is truly remarkable

I am humbled and grateful for the opportunity to share the knowledge and insights gathered in the creation of "ELU NATION." This book has been crafted with the utmost care and a genuine desire to empower you on your fitness journey. It is my sincerest hope that the contents within these pages provide you with the guidance and inspiration you need to reach your fitness goals.

Thank you for your trust in me as an author and coach. Your belief in the power of knowledge and your commitment to self-improvement reaffirm my passion for helping others. Your dedication to your health not only transforms your own life but serves as a beacon of inspiration for those around you.

I would also like to express my gratitude to the fitness community, which has provided invaluable support, camaraderie,and wisdom. Your passion for fitness and well-being creates a positive ripple effect, empowering countless individuals to strive for greatness.

Finally, a special thank you to my family, friends, and loved ones who have been unwavering pillars of support throughout this journey. Your encouragement, love, and understanding have fuled my determination to make a difference in the lives of others.

Remember, ELU NATION is not just a concept— it is acommunity built on shared values, perseverance, and a relentless pursuit of personal growth. Together, we can achieve greatness and a lasting impact on the world around us.

Thank You,

Lee

Resources

Growth Hormone and Obesity: https://pubmed.ncbi.nlm.nih.gov/32418587/

The Role of Growth Hormone in the Regulation of Protein Metabolism with Particular Reference to Conditions of Fasting: https://pubmed.ncbi.nlm.nih.gov/

Flipping the Metabolic Switch: Understanding and Applying the Health Benefits of Fasting: https://pubmed.ncbi.nlm.nih.gov/29086496/

Autophagy is required to maintain muscle: https://pubmed.ncbi.nlm.nih.gov/19945408/

Effect of Intermittent Fasting on Reproductive Hormone Levels in Females and Males: A Review of Human Trials(PCOS): https://pubmed.ncbi.nlm.nih.gov/35684143/https://pubmed.ncbi.nlm.nih.gov/35684143/

Protein Recommendations for Weight Loss in Elite Athletes: A Focus on Body Composition and Performance: https://pubmed.ncbi.nlm.nih.gov/29182451/

Regulation of gene expression by growth hormone: https://pubmed.ncbi.nlm.nih.gov/32151566/

Regulation of GH and GH Signaling Nutrients: https://pubmed.ncbi.nlm.nih.gov/34199514/

Growth hormone and protein metabolism:
https://pubmed.ncbi.nlm.nih.gov/19773097/

Darwin, sexual selection, and the brain:
https://pubmed.ncbi.nlm.nih.gov/33593899/

The impact of self-confidence on the compromise effect:
https://pubmed.ncbi.nlm.nih.gov/22512502/

Eating two larger meals a day (breakfast and lunch) is more effective than six smaller meals in a reduced-energy regimen for patients with type 2 diabetes: a randomised crossover study:
https://link.springer.com/article/10.1007/s00125-014-3253-5

Effects of Resistance Training Frequency on Measures of Muscle Hypertrophy: A Systematic Review and Meta-Analysis:
https://pubmed.ncbi.nlm.nih.gov/27102172/

Lifting Weights and Weight Loss:
https://uknow.uky.edu/research/new-uk-study-offers-insight-how-resistance-training-burns-fat